Why Am I Always Sick?

Breaking The Habits

Unveiling the Mystery of Getting Unnecessary Sick

Dr Sebastian Wayne

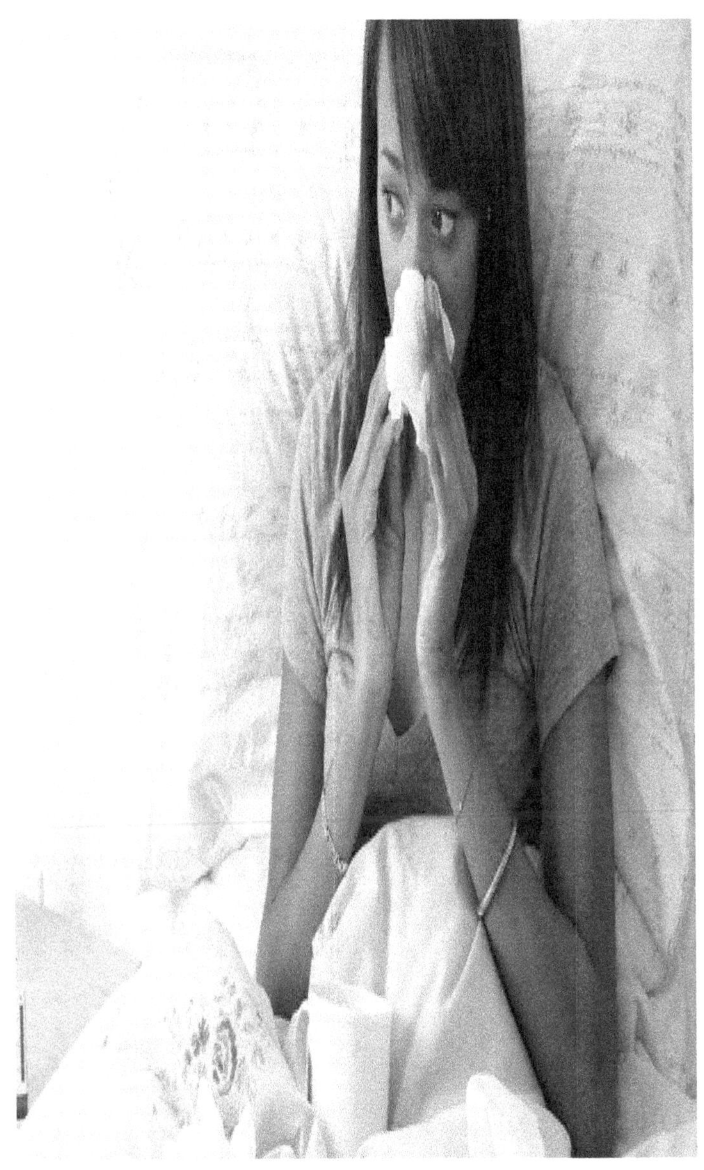

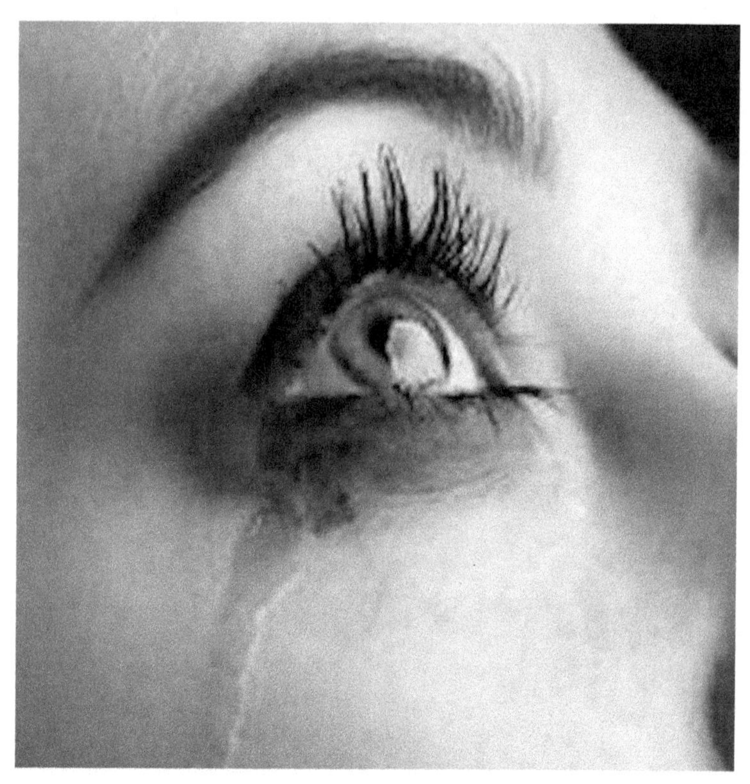

I AM SO SICK OF BEING SICK

CONTENTS

Cover page

CopyRight

Table Of Content

Introduction

Chapter 1

The Endless Cycle

Why I Am Always Sick

Lifestyles Changes To Boost Your Immune system

Chapter 2

Understanding The Body

Maintaining Our Health And Well Being

Factors Contributing To Our Health

Chapter 3

The Impact Of Lifestyles On Our Health

Understanding The Impact Of These Lifestyles

Lifestyle Changes For Wellness

Understanding Of The Factors Contributing To Your Persistence illness

Chapter 4

Mental And Emotional Well-being

Our Mental And Emotional State

Seeking Professional Guidance

Practical Guidance On Making Lifestyle Changes To Support Wellness

Actionable Steps You Can Take To Break Free From The Cycle Of Sickness

Introduction

Living with a chronic illness can be a difficult and stressful experience. Dealing with chronic illness can impact both your physical and mental health, from frequent colds and infections to persistent symptoms that seem to last for a long time. When you feel like you're constantly battling an illness, it's normal to feel irritable, anxious, and alone. Understanding the cause of your ongoing health problems is an important first step to relieving symptoms and improving your quality of life. Examining the root causes of common illnesses provides valuable insight into how to more effectively manage your health and make informed health decisions. This journey of self-discovery and empowerment will pave the way to better health and a brighter future.

CHAPTER 1

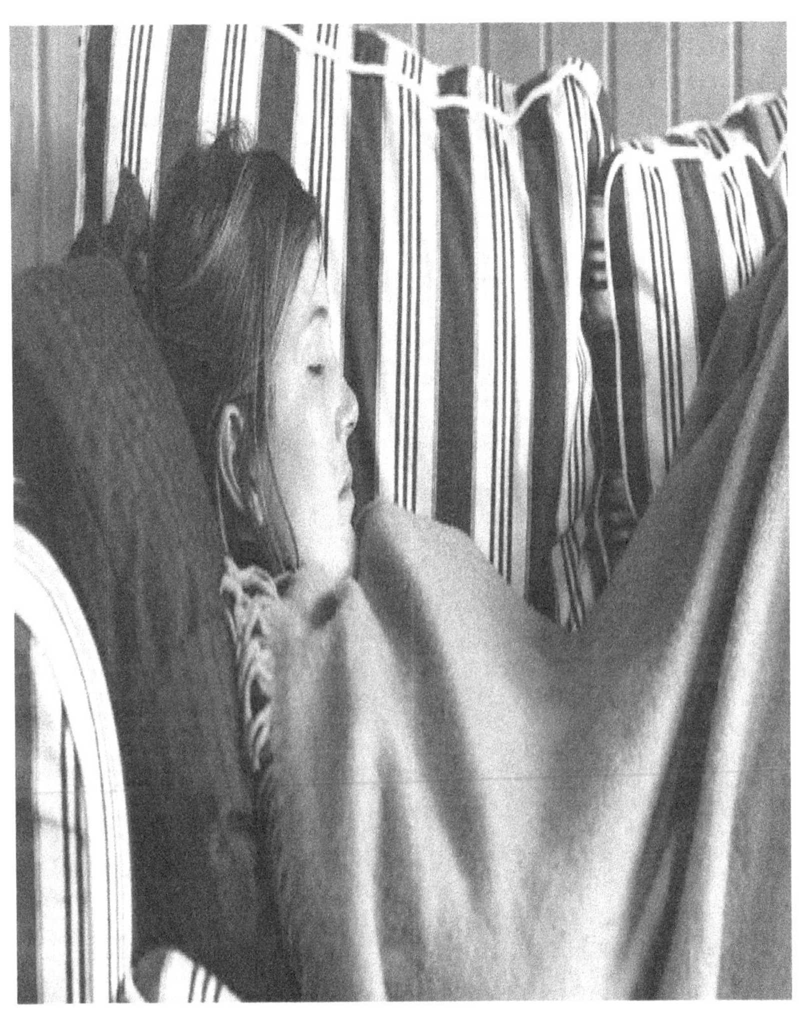

The Endless Cycle

Living with a   never-ending   cycle   of

constant illness can be an incredibly difficult and discouraging experience. It often feels like we are stuck in a never-ending cycle, where each illness flows seamlessly into the next, leaving us physically and mentally drained. This constant battle with your health can disrupt every aspect of your life, impacting your work, social life, and overall well-being.

One of the most frustrating aspects of this never-ending cycle is the feeling of not being able to fully recover until the next illness occurs. Just when you start to regain your strength and energy, you are hit by a wave of symptoms that return you to your illness again. This can lead to feelings of helplessness and frustration as you struggle to find peace and regain your health.

 The physical burden of ongoing illness is significant. Any   illness can weaken your immune system, making it   more difficult for your body to fight future infections. This creates a vicious cycle in which each disease further weakens your immune system, making you more likely to get sick again. In   addition, the physical   strain of ongoing illness can   cause   chronic fatigue, muscle weakness, and other physical symptoms that make daily life   difficult. Never underestimate the psychological impact of being constantly ill. Dealing with the frustration, disappointment, and anxiety that comes with chronic illness can take a toll on your mental health. It's not uncommon to feel isolated from friends and family who don't fully understand what you're going through, and the constant onslaught of illness can leave you feeling hopeless and hopeless. Over time, this can lead to depression and a general feeling of emotional exhaustion.

 Breaking out of the never-ending cycle of always being sick requires a multifaceted approach. Taking steps to support your immune system, treat underlying health issues, and change your lifestyle will go a long way in regaining control of your health.

An important first step is to work with your health care professional to identify any underlying health problems that may be making you more susceptible to the disease. This may require a thorough physical examination to rule out conditions such as autoimmune diseases, vitamin deficiencies, and chronic infections that can affect immune function. By addressing underlying health issues, you can take preventive measures to strengthen your immune system and reduce the incidence of disease.

In addition to treating underlying health issues, it's important to make lifestyle changes to support your overall health. This includes eating a nutritious diet, exercising regularly, getting enough sleep, and managing stress. A healthy lifestyle plays an important role in supporting immune function and reducing the risk of disease. Additionally, practicing good hygiene, such as washing hands frequently and avoiding contact with sick people, can help reduce exposure to pathogens and minimize the risk of illness.

Supporting your immune system with nutritional supplements and natural remedies can also be beneficial. Certain vitamins and minerals, such as vitamin C, zinc, and probiotics, have been shown to support immune function and may reduce the frequency and severity of illness. Herbal medicines and supplements such as echinacea, elderberry, and astragalus are also traditionally used to strengthen the immune system and support overall health.

Stress management techniques such as meditation, yoga, and breathing exercises play an important role in supporting overall health and immune function.

Chronic stress can negatively impact your immune system and make you more susceptible to illness. By incorporating stress reduction strategies into your daily life, you can reduce the impact of stress on your health and reduce your risk of disease.

Seeking support from friends, family, and support groups can also be very helpful in dealing with the ongoing challenges of a chronic illness. A strong support network provides emotional encouragement, practical assistance, and a sense of connectedness that can help you get through difficult times and maintain a positive attitude.

It's important to work closely with your doctor to develop an active plan for managing your health. This may include regular exams, monitoring key health indicators, and adjusting your treatment plan as necessary to address new or ongoing health concerns.

Living with a never-ending cycle of being sick all the time can be very difficult, but it's important to remember that there is hope for breaking out of this cycle. By taking a comprehensive approach to health care, addressing underlying issues, and making positive lifestyle changes, you can reduce your incidence of disease and regain your vitality. With patience, perseverance, and the right support, you can overcome the never-ending cycle of always being sick and move toward a healthier, more resilient future.

Why I am Always Sick

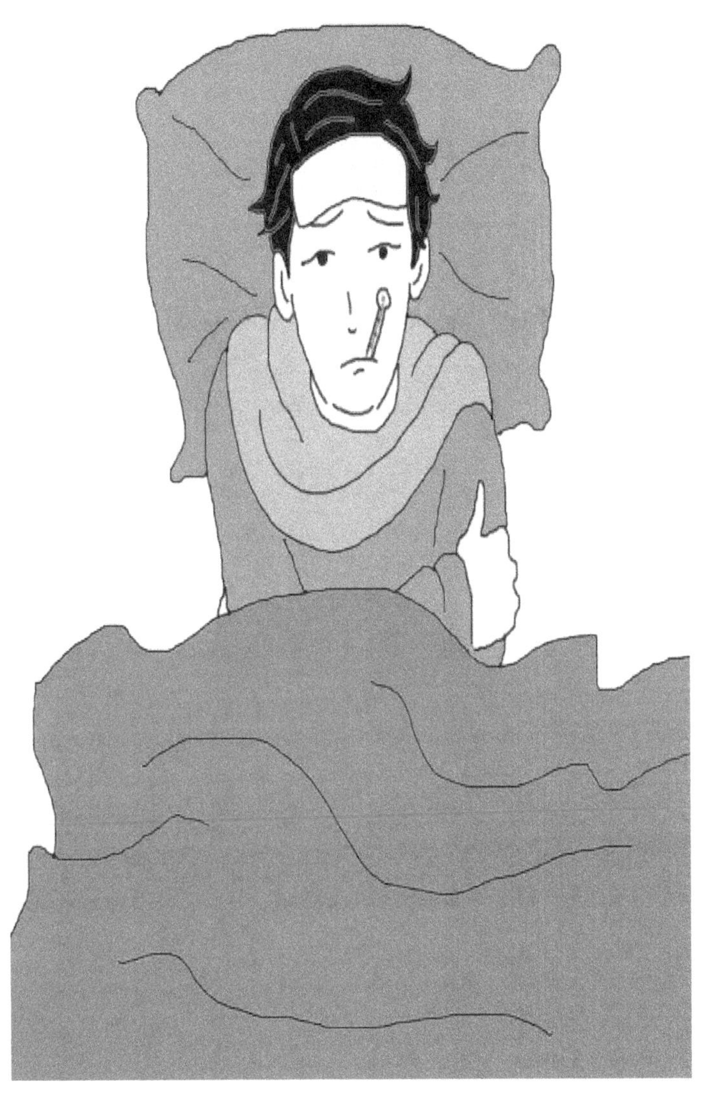

Common   illnesses can be frustrating and

worrying. There can be many reasons why someone gets sick often. Common causes include:

1. Weak immune system: If your immune system is not fully developed, as in young children, or if your immune system is weakened by certain medical conditions or treatments, you may be more susceptible to infections. .

2. Chronic conditions: Illnesses such as diabetes, asthma, and allergies can make you more susceptible to common illnesses.

3. Nutritional deficiencies: A diet lacking

essential vitamins and minerals can impair the immune system's ability to fight infections.

4. Stress: Chronic stress can weaken your immune system and make you more susceptible to illness.

5. Not enough sleep: Too little sleep affects your immune system and makes you more likely to get sick.

6. Poor hygiene: Improper hand washing and exposure to germs can lead to increased illness.

7. Environmental Factors: Exposure to allergens, pollutants, or toxic substances can cause health problems.

8. Sedentary lifestyle: Lack of regular

physical activity can weaken your immune system over time.

9. Age: Young children and older people tend to get sick more often because their immune systems develop or weaken with age. These factors are just illustrative of possible reasons. The exact cause of your particular situation needs to be evaluated by a doctor. Persistent or frequent illnesses may indicate an underlying health problem that requires proper diagnosis and treatment. If you are constantly suffering from an illness, it is important to consult a doctor to determine the cause and find the appropriate

treatment.

Improving sleep habits and overall lifestyle can indeed help boost your immune system. Here are some tips you can consider:

1. Establish a Regular Sleep Schedule: Aim to go to bed and wake up at the same time each day, even on weekends. This helps set your body's internal clock.

2. Create a peaceful environment: Keep your bedroom dark, quiet, and cool. Consider using blackout curtains, earplugs, and a white noise machine if needed.

3. Limit your screen time: Try to avoid

screens such as your phone, tablet, or computer at least an hour before bed. The blue light emitted can disrupt your sleep.

4. Watch your diet: Avoid heavy meals, caffeine, and alcohol close to bedtime. It can disrupt your sleep and reduce your sense of well-being.

5. Exercise regularly: Regular physical activity helps you fall asleep faster and get deeper sleep. However, avoid exercising too close to bedtime as it can have the opposite effect.

6. Manage stress: Practice relaxation techniques like deep breathing, meditation, and yoga. Managing stress

improves sleep quality and improves immune function.

7. Avoid naps: If you have trouble falling asleep at night, avoid naps during the day, especially in the afternoon.

8. Expose yourself to natural light: Spend time outdoors every day, especially in the morning, to help regulate your sleep-wake cycle.

9. Don't stay awake in bed: If you can't sleep, stay up and do something relaxing until you feel sleepy. Tossing and turning can create an unhealthy connection between your sleep environment and your wakefulness.

10. Consult a specialist: If your sleep

problems persist, we recommend that you consult your doctor or sleep specialist.

Lifestyle changes to boost your immune system:

1. Eat a balanced diet rich in fruits, vegetables, lean proteins, and whole grains to replenish essential nutrients.

2. Stay Hydrated: Drink plenty of water throughout the day.

3. Exercise: Aim for at least 150 minutes of moderate aerobic activity or 75 minutes of vigorous activity each week, plus strength training twice a week.

4. Limit your alcohol intake and quit smoking: Both can weaken your

immune system.

5. Maintain Good Hygiene: Washing your hands regularly helps prevent the spread of germs.

6. Regular Health Checks: Always receive vaccinations and regular health checkups.

Remember that lifestyle changes take time to adopt and should be approached realistically and sustainably. Gradual changes are more likely to become permanent parts of your lifestyle. Always consult with healthcare professionals when making significant changes to your health routine.

Managing stress is crucial for maintaining

mental and physical health. Here are some strategies and relaxation techniques that you can use:

1. Deep Breathing Exercises: Practice deep and slow breathing techniques such as the 4-7-8 method, where you inhale for 4 seconds, hold for 7 seconds, and exhale for 8 seconds. Deep breathing helps to reduce stress by activating the body's relaxation response.

2. Progressive Muscle Relaxation (PMR): Tense and then relax different muscle groups throughout your body, from your toes to your head. This technique helps relieve physical tension and stress.

3. Mindfulness and Meditation: Take time each day to practice mindfulness and meditation. Even a few minutes can help. Focus on being present in the moment and observe your thoughts and breathing without judgment.

4. Physical activity: Exercise is an effective stress reliever. Regular physical activity, such as a brisk walk, a gym workout, or a yoga class, can help reduce stress hormones, increase endorphins, and improve your mood.

5. Adequate sleep: Stress often disrupts sleep and creates a vicious cycle. Aim for 7 to 9 hours of quality sleep each night and follow good sleep hygiene

habits, including: For example, maintain a regular schedule, avoid screens before bed, and keep your bedroom comfortable and dark.

6. Healthy Eating: Eat a balanced diet rich in vegetables, fruits, lean proteins, and whole grains. Reduce your intake of caffeine and sugar, as they can worsen stress symptoms.

7. Time management: Prioritize tasks, break them down into manageable steps, and delegate when possible. Avoid procrastination and overcommitment. If you're already overloaded, learn how to say no to extra tasks.

8. Social care: Spend time with friends

and family. A support system provides mental peace and helps you get through stressful times.

9. Hobbies and interests: Participate in activities that are fun and relaxing. It can be anything, such as reading, gardening, painting, playing an instrument, etc.

10. Guided images and visualization: Imagine a calm and relaxing place. Using all five senses to imagine this environment in detail will put your mind in a more peaceful state.

11. Journaling: Writing down your

thoughts and feelings is a great way to reduce stress. This will allow you to process your emotions and may give you new insight into what is causing your stress.

12. Aromatherapy: Consider using essential oils or scented candles that promote relaxation, such as lavender, chamomile, or sandalwood.

13. Expert Support: If your stress feels overwhelming or persistent, you should consider consulting a mental health professional so that more individualized strategies and interventions can be developed. Keep in mind that different techniques

may be effective for different people, so it's important to find what works best for you. Try incorporating some of these strategies into your daily life and adjusting them as nccded. Regular practice makes a big difference in your stress levels and overall health.

CHAPTER 2

Understanding The Body

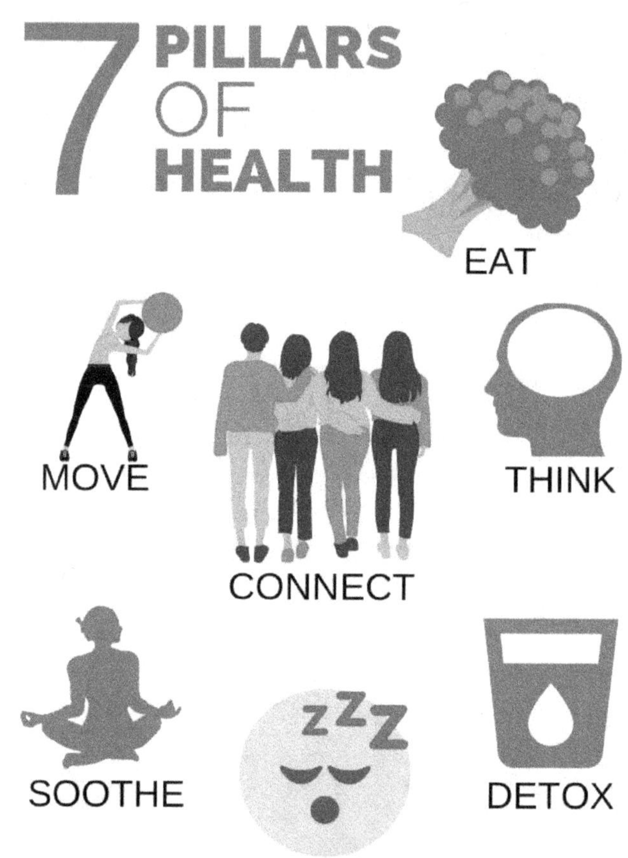

Understanding the human body requires an understanding of its anatomy and physiology and how its various systems work together to sustain life. From the intricate workings of the cardiovascular system to the complex interactions of hormones in the endocrine system, there is much to understand. Learning about the body's structure, function, and factors that influence health and well-being is important to a variety of fields, including medicine, biology, and health care. Understanding the human body involves several key aspects:

Anatomy: This refers to the structure of the body and its parts, including organs, tissues, cells, and their spatial relationships. It involves learning about bones, muscles, organs, blood vessels, nerves, and other structures, both externally and internally.

Physiology: Physiology focuses on the functions of these anatomical structures, how they work individually and together to maintain homeostasis (internal balance), and how they respond to various stimuli and environments. For example, understanding how the heart pumps blood, how the lungs exchange oxygen and carbon dioxide, and how the nervous system coordinates body activities.

Biochemistry: This area delves into the chemical processes and substances involved in the functioning of living organisms, including humans. It includes the study of molecules such as proteins, lipids, carbohydrates, and nucleic acids, as well as metabolic pathways and reactions within cells.

Pathophysiology: Pathophysiology explores the changes in physiological processes that occur due to disease, injury, or other abnormal conditions. It involves understanding how the body's systems are affected and how they respond to these disruptions, leading to the development of various health conditions.

Anatomical and physiological variations: Recognizing that there can be variations in anatomy and physiology among individuals due to factors such as genetics, age, gender, and environmental influences is also essential. These differences can influence how the disease manifests, how treatment is delivered, and how individuals respond to interventions. **Interconnection of Body Systems:** It is important to understand how the various systems within the body are connected and work together. For example, the cardiovascular system delivers oxygen and nutrients to tissues through blood vessels, the respiratory system supplies oxygen and removes carbon dioxide, and the digestive system processes nutrients for absorption.

Clinical relevance: Finally, understanding the human body is clinically important. Especially in fields such as medicine and healthcare. Medical professionals need a comprehensive understanding of anatomy and physiology to effectively diagnose and treat diseases, safely prescribe medications, and provide appropriate patient care.

However, anatomy and physiology play an important role in understanding disease, but in different ways.

1. Anatomy: Understanding the structure of the human body is important for diagnosing diseases and conditions.

Anatomical knowledge helps medical professionals detect abnormalities such as tumors, lesions, and structural defects through techniques such as physical examination, imaging (e.g., X-rays, MRI), and surgery. For example, determining the location and size of a tumor within an organ's anatomy is important in determining treatment options.

2. Physiology: Physiology provides information about how the body's systems function normally and how they are affected by illness and disease. Alterations in physiological processes underlie many diseases and disorders. For example, understanding how the immune system responds to pathogens can help diagnose infectious diseases, while knowledge of cardiovascular physiology is essential for treating conditions such as hypertension and heart failure.

Anatomy and physiology are both important, but physiology has a more direct impact on illness and disease because it deals with the functional aspects of the body and how they change in various pathological conditions. I often give. However, an understanding of anatomy is the basis for interpreting physiological changes and accurately diagnosing diseases. Therefore, both are essential in healthcare and medical practice.

Human anatomy is the study of the structure of the human body and its parts. It encompasses various levels of organization, from the smallest components of life to the entire body. Here's an overview of human anatomy and how it works.

1. Organizational level:

- Chemical level: At the smallest level, chemicals such as atoms and molecules form the building blocks of cells.

- Cellular Level: Cells are the basic structural and functional units of the body. They perform specific functions and vary in size, shape, and function.

- Tissue Level: A tissue is a group of similar cells that work together to perform a specific function. There are four main types of tissue: epithelial tissue, connective tissue, muscle tissue, and nervous tissue.

- Organ Level: Organs are made up of different types of tissues that work together to perform specific functions. Examples include the heart, lungs, liver, and brain.

- Organ system level: An organ system is a group of organs that work together to perform a coordinated function essential to the survival of an organism. Examples include the cardiovascular system, respiratory system, digestive system, nervous system, and skeletal system.

- Organizational Level: At the highest level, all organ systems work together to form the whole organism, the human body.

 2. Major organ systems:

- Skeletal system: Provides structural support, protects internal organs, and facilitates movement of bones and joints.

- Muscular system: Facilitates movement, maintains posture, generates heat, and supports other systems.

- Nervous System: Controls and coordinates the body's activities, processes sensory information, and allows communication between different parts of the body.

 - Cardiovascular system: Circulates blood throughout the body, delivering oxygen and nutrients while removing waste products.

-Respiratory System: Facilitates the exchange of oxygen and carbon dioxide between the body and the environment through breathing.

-Digestive system: Processes food, absorbs nutrients, and removes waste products.

- Endocrine system: Produces hormones that regulate various body functions and maintain homeostasis.   - **Immune system**:   Protects the body from pathogens and foreign substances and prevents infections and diseases.

- Integumentary System: protects the body from external attacks, regulates body temperature, and contains sensory receptors.

- Urinary system: Filters blood, removes waste products, and regulates electrolyte balance and fluid volume.

3. Functions of Human Anatomy:

- Support: Provides structural support and stability to the body.

- Protection: Protects vital organs from injury, damage, and pathogens.   - Movement: Facilitates movement through interactions between bones, muscles, and joints.

- Transportation: Transports nutrients, oxygen, waste products, and other substances throughout the body via blood and other bodily fluids.

- Homeostasis: Maintains internal balance and stability despite external changes.

-        Communication: Facilitates

communication between different parts of the body, allowing coordination and control of physical activity.

Understanding human anatomy is critical for medical professionals in diagnosing and treating diseases, performing surgeries, and providing effective patient care. This provides a foundation for understanding how the body works and how different systems interact to maintain health and well-being.

Human diseases and conditions can arise from a variety of anatomical factors, including structural abnormalities, organ and system dysfunction, and pathogen invasion. This is how anatomy plays a role in the development of disease.

1. Structural abnormalities: Anatomical variations or abnormalities can make people more susceptible to certain diseases or conditions. for example:

- Structural defects in organs and tissues, such as congenital heart defects, can lead to functional impairment and cardiovascular disease.

- Bone structure abnormalities such as scoliosis and kyphosis can cause musculoskeletal disorders and chronic pain.

- Anatomical differences in the airways,

such as: B. A deviated nasal septum and narrow airways can lead to respiratory diseases such as sleep apnea and chronic obstructive pulmonary disease (COPD).

2. Organ Malfunction: Disease can occur when an organ or system malfunctions due to anatomical abnormality or physiological malfunction.

- Impaired insulin production by the pancreas can lead to diabetes.

- Cirrhosis is caused by chronic liver damage, which destroys the organ's anatomy, impairs its function, and causes various complications.

3. Pathogen entry: Anatomical structures can serve as points of entry for pathogens, causing infections and disease.

- Bacteria and viruses can enter the body through wounds on the skin, mucous membranes, and respiratory and gastrointestinal tracts, causing infections such as pneumonia, urinary tract infections, and gastroenteritis.

- Anatomical structures such as the respiratory system are more susceptible to infections such as influenza and tuberculosis when airborne pathogens are inhaled.

4. Trauma and Injury: Anatomical

structures are susceptible to trauma and injury, which can lead to a variety of illnesses and conditions.

- Traumatic brain injury results from head trauma and can lead to neurological deficits and long-term complications. - Physical trauma can cause fractures and dislocations of bones and joints, leading to damage and dysfunction of the musculoskeletal system.

5. Tumor Growth: Abnormal growth or tumors develop within an anatomical structure and can disrupt its function and cause disease.

- Tumors can develop in organs such as

the lungs, liver, and colon, leading to diseases such as lung, liver, and colon cancer. - Even benign tumors can cause health problems if they grow in critical areas or put pressure on surrounding tissues or organs.

Understanding the anatomical basis of disease is important for effective diagnosis and treatment of disease. Medical professionals use their knowledge of human anatomy to detect abnormalities, assess the extent of disease, and develop appropriate treatment plans to restore health and well-being.

Human physiology is the branch of

biological science that focuses on how the human body functions at various levels of organization, from cellular and tissue levels to organ systems and the entire organism. It involves the study of the mechanisms and processes that occur within the body to maintain homeostasis, respond to internal and external stimuli, and sustain life.

Physiology explores how different systems and organs work together to perform specific functions necessary for survival and overall well-being. It encompasses a wide range of topics, including:Cellular Physiology: Examines the functions and activities of individual cells, including cellular metabolism, transport of substances across cell membranes, and cellular communication.Neurophysiology: Studies the function of the nervous system, including the generation and transmission of nerve impulses, synaptic transmission, and the integration of sensory information.

Cardiovascular Physiology: Focuses on the function of the heart and blood vessels, including the mechanisms of blood circulation, regulation of blood pressure, and cardiac output.

Respiratory Physiology: Investigates the processes involved in breathing, gas exchange in the lungs, transport of oxygen and carbon dioxide in the blood, and regulation of respiratory rate and depth.

Renal Physiology: Examines the function of the kidneys in maintaining fluid and electrolyte balance, regulating blood pressure, excreting waste products, and producing urine.

Endocrine Physiology: Studies the function of the endocrine system, including hormone secretion, regulation of metabolic processes, and coordination of various physiological functions.

Gastrointestinal Physiology: Focuses on the processes of digestion, absorption of nutrients, secretion of digestive enzymes and hormones, and regulation of gastrointestinal motility.

Muscle Physiology: Investigates the function of skeletal, smooth, and cardiac muscles, including muscle contraction, energy metabolism, and the role of muscles in movement and thermoregulation.

Immune Physiology: Examines the function of the immune system in defending the body against pathogens, including the cellular and molecular mechanisms of immune responses.

Reproductive Physiology: Studies the function of the male and female reproductive systems, including gametogenesis, hormone regulation of reproductive cycles, fertilization, pregnancy, and childbirth.

Human sickness or illness can occur due to various physiological factors, which involve the malfunctioning or disruption of normal bodily processes, Here's how physiology plays a role in causing sickness.

Homeostatic Imbalance: Homeostasis refers to the body's ability to maintain a stable internal environment despite external changes. When there is a disruption in homeostasis, it can lead to sickness.

For example: Temperature Regulation: If the body fails to regulate its temperature properly, it can lead to heat stroke or hypothermia.

Fluid and Electrolyte Balance: Imbalances in fluid and electrolyte levels can lead to conditions like dehydration or electrolyte disturbances.

Dysregulation of Physiological Processes: Malfunctions in physiological processes can result in various illnesses.

Endocrine Disorders: Dysregulation of hormone secretion and action can lead to conditions like diabetes mellitus, thyroid disorders, or adrenal insufficiency.

Cardiovascular Disorders: Dysfunction in the cardiovascular system can lead to hypertension, heart failure, arrhythmias, or atherosclerosis.

Respiratory Disorders: Dysfunction in the respiratory system can lead to conditions like asthma, chronic obstructive pulmonary disease (COPD), or respiratory infections.

Renal Disorders: Dysfunction in the kidneys can lead to conditions like kidney stones, urinary tract infections, or renal failure.Genetic Factors: Genetic variations or mutations can predispose individuals to certain physiological disorders or diseases.

For example, Cystic Fibrosis: A genetic mutation leads to abnormal function of the CFTR protein, affecting the lungs, pancreas, and other organs.

Sickle Cell Disease: Genetic mutation in hemoglobin leads to abnormal red blood cells, causing vaso-occlusive crises and other complications.Infections and Inflammation: Pathogens such as bacteria, viruses, fungi, or parasites can disrupt normal physiological processes, leading to sickness,

Infectious Diseases: Pathogens can infect various tissues and organs, leading to illnesses like pneumonia, influenza, gastroenteritis, or urinary tract infections.

Inflammatory Disorders: Dysregulated immune responses can lead to chronic inflammation and autoimmune diseases like rheumatoid arthritis, lupus, or inflammatory bowel disease.

Environmental Factors: Environmental exposures can affect physiological function and contribute to sickness.

Toxic Exposures: Exposure to toxins or pollutants can disrupt physiological processes and lead to conditions like poisoning or organ damage.

Allergens: Exposure to allergens can trigger abnormal immune responses, leading to allergic reactions like asthma or allergic rhinitis.

Lifestyle Factors: Poor lifestyle choices or behaviors can impact physiological function and contribute to sickness.

Diet and Nutrition: Poor diet can lead to nutrient deficiencies or metabolic disorders like obesity or diabetes.Physical Activity: Lack of exercise can contribute to cardiovascular diseases, obesity, or musculoskeletal disorders.Substance Abuse: Substance abuse can affect physiological function and contribute to conditions like liver disease, cardiovascular disorders, or neurological disorders.

Maintaining Our Health And Well-

being

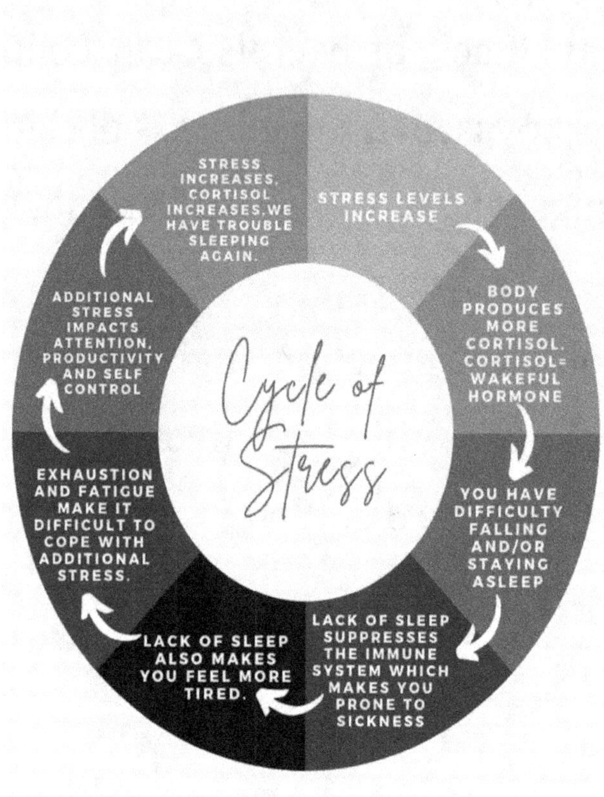

Maintaining our health and well-being is

vital to living a happy and fulfilling life. Key aspects to pay attention to are:

1. Balanced diet:

- Eat a variety of foods to get all the nutrients you need.

- Focus on whole grains, fruits, vegetables, lean proteins, and healthy fats.

- Limit your intake of processed foods, sugar, and saturated fat.

2. Regular exercise:

- Aim for at least 150 minutes of moderate aerobic activity or 75 minutes of vigorous activity per week.

- Include strength training at least twice a

week.

- Be consistent and find activities you enjoy.

 three.

3. Hydration:

 - Drink plenty of water throughout the day.

- Limit sugary drinks and excessive caffeine intake.

 4. Dream:

 - Aim for 7 to 9 hours of quality sleep per night.

- Establish comfortable sleeping habits.

- Maintain a consistent sleep schedule.

5. Mental Health:

- Practice stress-reduction techniques such as meditation, yoga, or deep breathing exercises.

- Connect with friends and family for social support.

- If you feel burdened or burdened, get help from a professional.

6. Preventive Healthcare:

- Get regular checkups, examinations, and vaccinations.

- Pay attention to your body and don't ignore warning signs.

7. Healthy Habits:

- Avoid smoking and limit drinking.

- Maintain good hygiene and wash your hands frequently.

- Be careful of ultraviolet rays. Use sunscreen and wear protective clothing.

8. Work-life balance:

- Take regular breaks while working.

- Set aside time for relaxation and hobbies.

- Learn to say "no" to excessive time wasters.

9. Mindfulness and Relaxation:

- Spend time doing relaxing activities such as reading, painting, or gardening. - Practice mindfulness to stay present and reduce stress.

10. Continuing Education:

- Challenge your brain by solving puzzles, reading or learning new skills.

- Remain curious and interested in the world around you.

By incorporating these practices into your daily life, you can significantly improve your health and overall well-being. Remember that small, incremental changes can have a big impact over time. Always consult a healthcare professional for tailored advice and support.

Factors Contribute To Our Health

PHYSICAL
healthy eating
personal hygiene
exercise
fun physical activity
regular sleep
medical check-up
physical appearance
rest after work
rest when sick
go for a walk

PSYCHOLOGICAL
practice a hobby
learn something new
read
challenge yourself
do something creative
no-screen hour
alone time
delayed gratification
go on a day-trip
practice patience

EMOTIONAL
time with loved ones
reflect
express feelings
feel the feelings
laugh
affirmations
respect yourself
stress management
talk about problems

SPIRITUAL
meditate
pray
find meaning
priorities and values
stand by your morals
contemplate life
think about mortality
observe your thoughts
participate in a cause

SOCIAL
time with loved ones
stay in contact
meaningful dialogue
have fun together
take a trip together
ask and offer help
meet new people
smile to a stranger
be polite

PROFESSIONAL
stay in the loop
work on your skills
read relevant literature
get involved
prevent burnout
organize workspace
plan the work
work on relationships

Health is a complex and multifaceted concept that is influenced by many factors.

The main participants are:

1. Genetics. Genetic predisposition can play an important role in an individual's health and affect their risk of developing certain diseases and conditions.

2. Diet. Nutrition is very important. A balanced intake of vitamins, minerals, fiber, protein, and other nutrients is essential to staying healthy.

3. Physical activity. Regular exercise promotes cardiovascular health, muscle development, flexibility, weight control, and mental health.

4. Dream. Adequate, quality sleep is vital for recovery, memory strengthening, and

hormonal balance.

5. Hydration. Water is essential for almost all body functions, including digestion, circulation, and temperature regulation.

6. Mental health. Stress, anxiety, depression, and other mental disorders have a huge impact on your overall well-being.

7. Social Connection. Support from friends and family can provide emotional support and reduce feelings of loneliness and isolation.

8. Access to health care. Availability and accessibility to health care services allow

health problems to be identified and treated early.

9. Environment. Clean air, safe drinking water, and a safe environment are the foundations of good health.

10. Lifestyle Choice. Smoking, drinking, and drug use can have serious negative effects on your health.

11. Education and Awareness. Understanding health risks and knowing how to manage them can help people make healthier choices.

12. Economic Power. Financial stability can affect access to nutritious food,

healthcare, and living conditions that promote a healthy lifestyle.

13. Occupation: Some occupations carry risks that can affect your health, while others may affect your health by promoting a sedentary lifestyle.

14. Cultural traditions. Cultural norms can influence diet, activity levels, and access to medical care.

15. Psychological state. Attitudes and worldviews can influence behavior and physiological health. For example, optimism and resilience are associated with improved health outcomes.

Balancing these factors is part of

maintaining good health. It's important to consider how each factor affects your life and what changes you can make to improve your overall well-being.

Here are some effective stress reduction techniques to try:

1. Mindfulness Meditation. Sit in a quiet place, focus on your breathing, and bring your attention back to the present moment when your mind wanders.

2. Deep breath. Practice slow, deep breathing techniques like the 4-7-8 method to calm your nervous system.

3.   Progressive   Muscle   Relaxation:

Relieves physical tension by alternately tensing and relaxing multiple muscle groups.

4. Regular exercise. Physical activity increases endorphins and helps relieve stress by providing relief from everyday worries.

 5. Yoga. It combines physical movement, meditation, gentle exercise, and controlled breathing to provide excellent stress relief.

6. Aromatherapy: Use essential oils like lavender, sandalwood, or orange blossom, which may have a calming effect.

7. Nature Time: Spend time outdoors.

Natural scenery and fresh air can help lower stress levels.

8. Guided Imagination. Visualize peaceful images and scenes that relax your mind.

9. Tai Chi or Qigong. This gentle form of martial arts helps balance and calm the mind through slow, deliberate movements and deep breathing.

10. Art and Music Therapy: Participate in creative activities such as painting or listening to soothing music.

11. Leading. Writing down your thoughts can provide you with an opportunity to express and understand your feelings.

12. Time Management. Organize your

schedule to avoid confusion that can lead to stress.

13. Social Interaction. Spend time with friends and loved ones to boost your mood and distract you from stressors.

14. Laughter Yoga. Join a laughter yoga class to relieve stress through fun and exciting activities that make you laugh.

15. Healthy Boundaries: Learn how to say "no" to requests that can be time-consuming and cause undue stress.

16. Treatment or Counseling. Talk to a mental health professional to learn how to manage stress and reduce its emotional impact.

17. Mindful eating. Eat slowly and enjoy your food. This helps reduce stress related to food and digestion. Try a few of the following techniques to see which one works best for you. The key is regular practice. Even just a few minutes a day can make a significant difference in reducing your stress levels.

CHAPTER 3

The Impact of Lifestyle

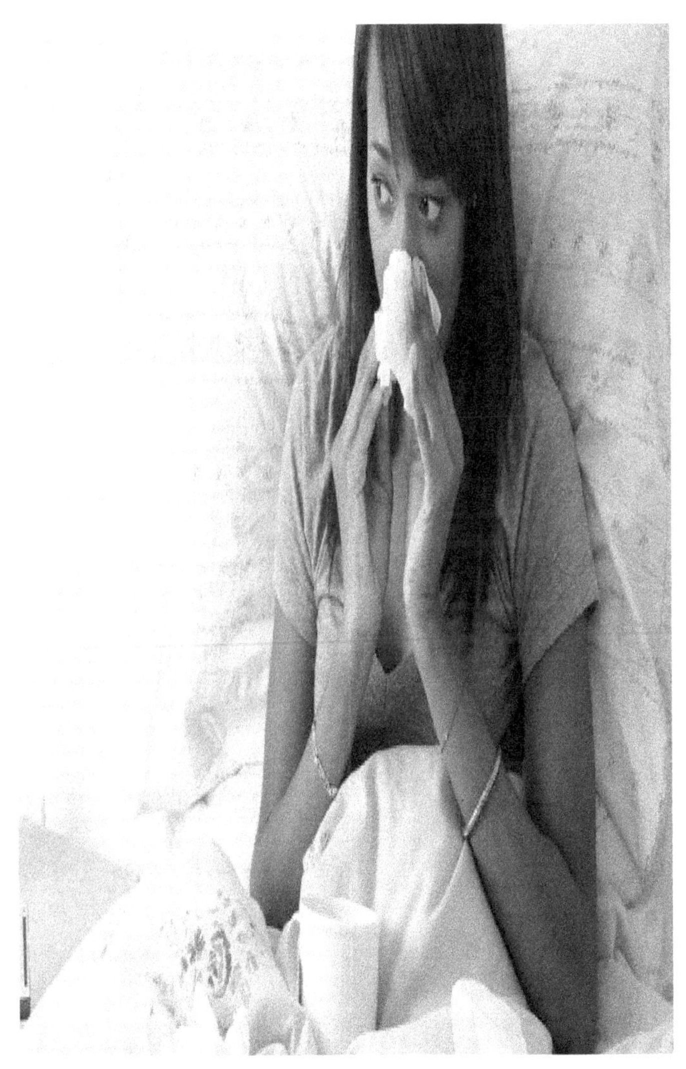

Human health is influenced by various factors, among which lifestyle plays a decisive role. Lifestyle includes the daily habits, behaviors, and choices an individual makes, including diet, physical activity, sleep patterns, stress management, and medication use. The impact of lifestyle on health is profound and far-reaching, affecting both physical and mental well-being. In this article, we will look at various aspects of lifestyle and how it affects a person's health.

Diet and Nutrition:

One of the most important factors affecting your overall health is diet and nutrition. A balanced diet rich in fruits, vegetables, whole grains, and lean proteins provides essential nutrients and antioxidants necessary for bodily functions. Conversely, a diet high in processed foods, saturated fats, sugars, and sodium increases the risk of obesity, cardiovascular diseases, diabetes, and certain cancers. Making informed food choices and practicing portion control are vital for maintaining optimal health.

Physical Activity:

Regular physical activity is crucial for maintaining a healthy weight, strengthening muscles and bones, improving cardiovascular health, and reducing the risk of chronic diseases.

Sedentary lifestyles characterized by prolonged sitting or lack of exercise contribute to obesity, heart disease, stroke, type 2 diabetes, and depression. Incorporating aerobic exercises, strength training, and flexibility exercises into daily routines can significantly enhance physical and mental well-being.

Sleep Patterns:

Quality sleep is essential for overall health and functioning. Adequate sleep duration and quality impact immune function, cognitive performance, mood regulation, and metabolic processes. Poor sleep hygiene, including irregular sleep schedules, excessive screen time before bedtime, and sleep disorders, such as insomnia and sleep apnea, can lead to fatigue, impaired concentration, weight gain, and increased risk of chronic diseases. Establishing a consistent sleep schedule and creating a relaxing bedtime routine are key components of good sleep hygiene.

Stress Management:

Chronic stress can have detrimental effects on health, contributing to hypertension, immune system dysfunction, digestive disorders, and mental health conditions like anxiety and depression. Effective stress management techniques, such as mindfulness meditation, deep breathing exercises, regular physical activity, and maintaining a strong social support network, can help mitigate the negative impact of stress on health.

Substance Use:

The consumption of tobacco, alcohol, and illicit drugs significantly impacts health outcomes. Tobacco smoking is a leading cause of preventable diseases, including lung cancer, cardiovascular diseases, and respiratory conditions. Excessive alcohol consumption increases the risk of liver disease, cardiovascular problems, and mental health disorders. Illicit drug use can lead to addiction, overdose, and various health complications. Adopting healthy coping mechanisms and seeking support for substance use disorders are essential for preserving health and well-being.

lifestyle choices profoundly influence human health and well-being. Adopting healthy habits related to diet, physical activity, sleep, stress management, and substance use can significantly improve health outcomes and quality of life. By making informed choices and prioritizing behaviors conducive to good health, individuals can empower themselves to lead fulfilling and vibrant lives. Remember that small changes to your lifestyle can have significant benefits for your long-term health and happiness.

Bad Habits such as smoking is very unhealthy as it may damage body organs such as lungs, livers and heart, how do I quite such bad Habits quitting smoking is a great decision for your health and well-being, albeit a challenging one. Here's an abridged action plan to help you quit successfully:

Commit and Set a Date

Commit to the decision to quit and set a quit date, preferably within the next two weeks. This gives you enough time to prepare without losing your motivation.

Understand Your Triggers

Identify what prompts you to smoke, such as stress, social activities, or after meals, and plan alternatives for those triggers.

Prepare to Manage Withdrawal

Expect withdrawal symptoms such as irritability, cravings, and difficulty concentrating. Plan strategies to cope, such as deep breathing, exercise, or engaging in hobbies.

Use Stop-Smoking Aids

Consider nicotine replacement therapy (NRT) like patches, gum, or lozenges, or prescription medications. Consult with a healthcare professional about these options.

Get Support

Inform friends and family of your plan to quit; their support can make a big difference. Also, consider joining support groups or online forums.

Practice Mindfulness and Relaxation Techniques

Mindfulness can reduce the intensity of cravings. Techniques such as yoga, meditation, or Tai Chi can help manage stress and improve your mental resilience.

Lifestyle Changes

Make healthy lifestyle changes that

reinforce your decision to quit. Exercise regularly, eat a balanced diet, and ensure you get enough sleep.

Avoid High-Risk Situations

Alcohol, parties, or friends who smoke can increase the temptation to smoke. Avoid these high-risk situations, especially in the early stages of quitting.

Reward Yourself

Set up a reward system for your milestones (1 day, 1 week, 1 month, etc.). Use the money you save from not buying cigarettes to treat yourself.

Create New Routines

Replace the habit of smoking with healthier habits. If you smoked with your morning coffee, try tea instead. If you took breaks to smoke, walk instead.

Stay Positive

Quitting is tough, and slips can happen. Don't be too hard on yourself if you have a cigarette. Regroup and focus on what led to the slip so you can prevent it in the future.

Continuous Learning

Read books, watch videos, and educate yourself about the benefits of quitting smoking and the risks of continuing.

Seek Professional Help

Professionals like doctors, therapists, or counselors can provide personalized support and strategies, especially if you're struggling with anxiety or depression. Remember that quitting is a journey— some days will be harder than others. Each day without a cigarette is a victory, and over time, it'll get easier. Stick with it.

Here's a detailed explanation of the impact of lifestyle on the frequency of illnesses, Poor dietary habits, such as consuming excessive processed foods, sugary snacks, and unhealthy fats, can weaken the immune system, leaving individuals more susceptible to illnesses. Conversely, a balanced diet rich in fruits, vegetables, whole grains, and lean proteins provides essential nutrients and antioxidants necessary to support immune health and reduce the risk of frequent illnesses.Sedentary lifestyles contribute to weakened immunity by reducing blood circulation and impairing immune cell function. Regular exercise enhances immune function by promoting better circulation, increasing the production of immune cells, and reducing inflammation. Engaging in moderate-intensity exercise for at least 30 minutes most days of the week can strengthen the immune system and lower the frequency of illnesses.Inadequate or poor-quality sleep disrupts the body's natural immune response, leaving individuals more susceptible to infections. Chronic sleep deprivation suppresses immune function and increases the risk of illnesses such as colds, flu, and respiratory infections. Prioritizing sufficient and restorative sleep supports optimal immune function, reducing the likelihood of frequent illnesses.Chronic stress triggers the release of stress hormones, which can suppress immune function and increase vulnerability to infections. Prolonged stress weakens the body's ability to fight off pathogens, leading to more frequent illnesses and slower recovery times. Implementing stress-reduction techniques such as mindfulness, deep breathing exercises, and regular relaxation practices can help strengthen the immune system and reduce the frequency of illnesses.Poor hygiene habits, such as inadequate handwashing and sanitation, facilitate the transmission of pathogens and increase the risk of infections. Proper hand hygiene, including washing hands with soap and water for at least 20 seconds, helps prevent the spread of germs and reduces the likelihood of contracting illnesses. Practicing good hygiene in personal and environmental settings can significantly decrease the frequency of illnesses by minimizing exposure to pathogens.Excessive alcohol consumption and smoking weaken the immune system, making individuals more susceptible to infections and illnesses. Substance abuse can impair immune function and compromise overall health, increasing the risk of frequent illnesses. Avoiding harmful substances and adopting healthy lifestyle choices can strengthen the immune system and reduce the frequency of illnesses.Environmental pollutants and toxins can compromise immune function and increase susceptibility to infections and illnesses. Poor air quality, exposure to allergens, and environmental hazards contribute to respiratory problems and other health issues. Minimizing exposure to environmental toxins and pollutants through measures such as air purification, proper ventilation, and avoidance of allergens can help reduce the frequency of illnesses.In summary, lifestyle choices profoundly impact the frequency of illnesses by either strengthening or weakening the immune system. Adopting healthy habits related to diet, exercise, sleep, stress management, hygiene, and substance use can significantly reduce the likelihood of getting sick frequently, leading to improved overall health and well-being.

Understanding The Impact Of These

Lifestyle

Lifestyle generally refers to the lifestyle of an individual or group. It includes habits, attitudes, tastes, moral standards, economic standards and social norms that together shape the daily life of an individual or community. Some key aspects that are often included in lifestyle discussions include:

1. Health and Wellness Habits related to physical health (exercise, diet), mental health, stress management and medical practice.

2. Leisure and recreation Activities performed for pleasure during leisure time, such as hobbies, sports, or cultural

events.

3. Work-life balance. How people manage their time and focus on their professional responsibilities and personal life.

4. Consumption Pattern. The way people acquire, use, and dispose of goods and services reflects their economic status and personal values.

5. Social Life The extent and nature of a person's interactions with family, friends, and society.

6. Environmental Impact: The impact of human lifestyles on the environment, taking into account sustainability and ecological footprint.

Lifestyle is influenced by a variety of factors, including income, education, religion, culture, and physical environment, and often changes over time. Understanding lifestyles can help you develop products, services, and policies that meet the needs and desires of different groups.

Lifestyle encompasses the daily habits, behaviors, and choices individuals make, influencing their health and well-being. These choices, including diet, physical activity, sleep patterns, stress management, substance use, hygiene practices, and social interactions, significantly impact susceptibility to illnesses and chronic diseases. Certain lifestyles contribute to poor health outcomes:

Poor Dietary Habits: Excessive consumption of processed foods, sugary snacks, and unhealthy fats while lacking essential nutrients weakens the immune system and increases the risk of chronic diseases like obesity, diabetes, and heart disease.

Sedentary Lifestyle: Lack of regular physical activity and prolonged sitting increase the risk of obesity, cardiovascular diseases, diabetes, and weakened immunity, making individuals more susceptible to illnesses.Inadequate Sleep: Insufficient sleep or poor sleep quality impairs immune function, increases stress levels, and raises the risk of infections, mental health issues, and chronic diseases.Chronic Stress: Prolonged exposure to stress hormones weakens the immune system, leading to increased susceptibility to infections, inflammation, and chronic conditions such as hypertension, diabetes, and depression.

Poor Hygiene Practices: Neglecting proper

handwashing, sanitation, and hygiene increases the risk of infectious diseases and illnesses caused by bacteria, viruses, and other pathogens.Substance Abuse: Excessive consumption of alcohol, tobacco, and illicit drugs weakens immune function, impairs organ health, and increases susceptibility to infections, respiratory problems, and chronic diseases.

Developing Good Lifestyles for Better Health:To promote health and well-being, individuals can adopt the following strategies:Healthy Eating: Focus on a balanced diet rich in fruits, vegetables, whole grains, lean proteins, and healthy fats. Limit processed foods, sugary snacks, and unhealthy fats.Regular Exercise: Incorporate regular physical activity into daily routines, including aerobic exercises, strength training, and flexibility exercises. Aim for at least 150 minutes of moderate-intensity exercise per week.

Adequate Sleep: Prioritize sufficient and restorative sleep by maintaining a consistent sleep schedule, creating a relaxing bedtime routine, and ensuring a comfortable sleep environment.Stress Management: Practice stress-reduction techniques such as mindfulness meditation, deep breathing exercises, yoga, and relaxation techniques to manage stress levels effectively.

Hygiene Practices: Maintain good hygiene by washing hands regularly with soap and water, practicing proper food handling and sanitation, and maintaining cleanliness in personal and environmental settings.

Avoiding Harmful Substances: Limit or avoid excessive alcohol consumption, tobacco smoking, and illicit drug use to protect immune function, organ health, and overall well-being.Social Support: Cultivate strong social connections and supportive relationships to promote emotional well-being, reduce stress, and enhance overall health.In conclusion, lifestyle choices significantly impact human health and well-being. By adopting a healthy lifestyle, people can live happier, more satisfying lives by improving their health, strengthening their immune system, and reducing their risk of illness and chronic disease.

Lifestyle Changes for Wellness

Lifestyle changes for wellness refer to intentional modifications in daily habits, behaviors, and choices aimed at improving overall well-being and promoting a healthy lifestyle. These changes encompass various aspects of life, including diet, physical activity, sleep patterns, stress management, social interactions, and self-care practices. The goal of lifestyle changes for wellness is to optimize physical, mental, and emotional health, leading to a higher quality of life and greater longevity.

Key components of lifestyle changes for wellness include:

1. Healthy Eating: Adopting a balanced diet rich in fruits, vegetables, whole grains, lean proteins, and healthy fats while minimizing processed foods, sugary snacks, and unhealthy fats. Paying attention to portion sizes and mindful eating can also contribute to overall wellness.

2. Regular Exercise: Incorporating regular physical activity into daily routines, including aerobic exercises, strength training, flexibility exercises, and

activities that promote movement and mobility. Aim for at least 150 minutes of moderate-intensity exercise per week to improve cardiovascular health, muscle strength, and overall fitness.

3. Adequate Sleep: Prioritize adequate, restorative sleep by maintaining a consistent sleep schedule, establishing comfortable sleep habits, and creating a comfortable sleep environment. Quality sleep is essential for physical recovery, cognitive function, mood regulation, and overall well-being.

4. Stress Management: Use stress reduction techniques such as mindfulness

meditation, deep breathing exercises, progressive muscle relaxation, yoga, and other relaxation techniques. Finding healthy coping mechanisms and effective stress management strategies can promote emotional resilience and mental well-being.

5. Social Connections: Develop strong social connections and supportive relationships with family, friends, and community members. Being socially active, participating in group activities, and seeking social support can improve emotional well-being, reduce loneliness, and improve overall quality of life.

6. Practice self-care. Prioritize self-care activities that promote physical, mental, and emotional health, such as practicing gratitude, engaging in hobbies and interests, spending time outdoors, and making time for rest and relaxation. . Holistic self-care is essential to your overall well-being.

7. Mind-Body Practices: Integrate mind-body practices such as yoga, tai chi, qigong, and meditation into your daily life to promote relaxation, stress reduction, and mind-body awareness. These practices can help improve physical health, mental clarity, and emotional balance.

Through conscious lifestyle changes that prioritize health, people can improve their overall health, vitality, and quality of life. Consistency and commitment to these changes are key to reaping long-term benefits and achieving optimal well-being.

There are many factors that influence lifestyle changes and can vary depending on your individual circumstances and goals. Some key factors that typically influence lifestyle changes include:

1. Health Concerns Personal health concerns, such as a chronic disease diagnosis, symptoms associated with a poor lifestyle, or a desire to prevent future health problems, can motivate people to

make positive lifestyle changes.

2. Family and Social Support Support from family, friends or social networks can play an important role in lifestyle changes. Encouragement, accountability, and sharing can help people stay motivated and committed to their goals.

3. Knowledge and Education Access to information and education about the importance of a healthy lifestyle, understanding the risks associated with unhealthy behaviors, and learning effective strategies for making positive changes can help people live healthier lives. It can empower you to live .

4. Environmental factors, such as access to healthy food, opportunities for physical activity, access to health care, and community resources, can affect people's ability to change their lifestyles. A supportive environment that promotes healthy behaviors can promote positive change.

5. Personal Motivation and Goals Personal motivation, including internal factors such as the desire to feel better, increase energy levels, and improve quality of life, or external factors such as appearance or performance goals, helps people make changes. It can motivate you to do it. lifestyle.

6. Cultural and Social Influences Cultural norms, social expectations and social norms regarding health and lifestyle can influence people's choices and behavior. Cultural customs, traditions, and beliefs can also shape attitudes toward certain lifestyle habits.

7. Economic Considerations Economic factors such as financial resources, availability of healthy food, availability of recreational facilities, and availability of health care can affect people's ability to change their lifestyle. Socioeconomic status can affect access to resources that support healthy behavior.

8. Psychological Factors Psychological factors, including self-efficacy, self-discipline, resilience and coping skills, play an important role in people's ability to initiate and maintain lifestyle changes. Positive thinking, goal setting, and problem-solving skills are important to overcome problems and setbacks.

9. Life Changes and Events Life changes, such as starting a new job, moving to a new location, becoming a parent, or experiencing a significant life event, can create opportunities or challenges for lifestyle changes. This transition may cause people to rethink their priorities and adjust their lifestyles.

10. Peer Influence and Social Norms: Social influence from peers, colleagues, or social networks can influence an individual's lifestyle choices. Social support, encouragement, or peer pressure to adopt certain behaviors can influence people's decisions to change their lifestyle.

Typically, lifestyle changes are influenced by a combination of personal, social, environmental, and psychological factors. Understanding these factors can help people identify barriers to change, leverage enablers, and develop effective strategies for sustainable lifestyle change.

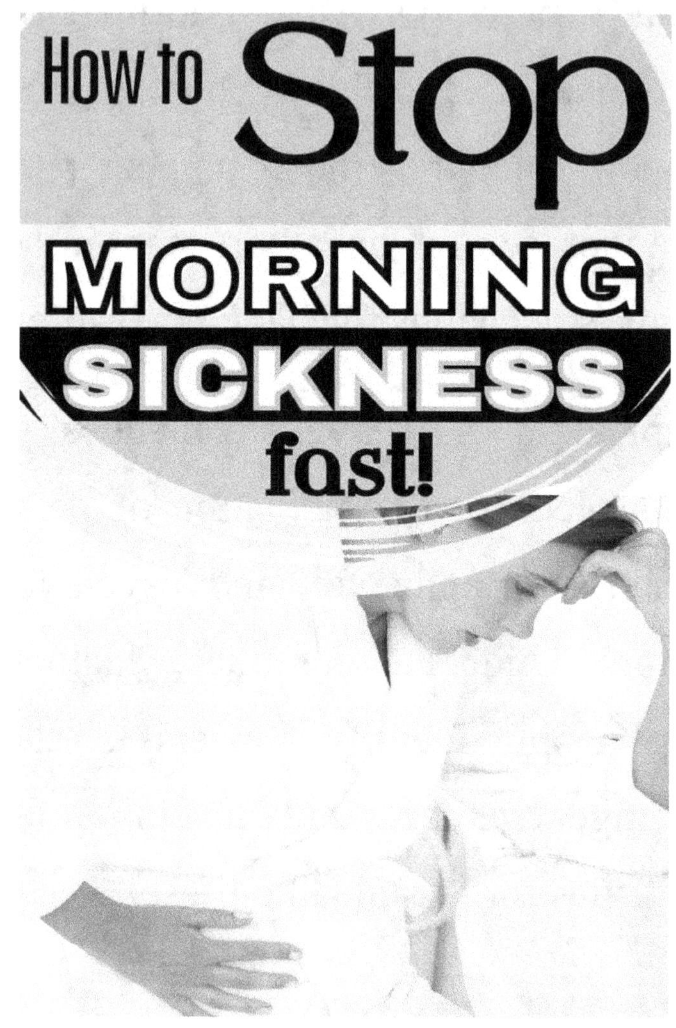
How to Stop
MORNING
SICKNESS
fast!

Persistent illness refers to a health condition or disease that continues over an extended period, often despite treatment or intervention. These illnesses typically last for weeks, months, or even years and may require ongoing management or treatment. Examples of persistent illnesses include chronic conditions such as diabetes, hypertension, asthma, autoimmune disorders, mental health disorders, and certain types of cancer. These conditions can significantly impact an individual's quality of life and may require long-term medical care, lifestyle modifications, and support to manage symptoms and prevent complications.

Persistent illness encompasses a wide range of health conditions that persist over time, impacting individuals physically, emotionally, and socially. These illnesses may vary in severity, duration, and management strategies, but they share the common characteristic of lasting beyond the acute phase.Examples of persistent illnesses include:

Chronic Conditions: Conditions such as diabetes, hypertension, heart disease, chronic obstructive pulmonary disease (COPD), and arthritis are characterized by long-term management and may require ongoing medication, lifestyle modifications, and regular medical monitoring.

Autoimmune Disorders: Autoimmune diseases like rheumatoid arthritis, lupus, multiple sclerosis, and inflammatory bowel disease involve the immune system attacking healthy tissues, leading to chronic inflammation and symptoms that persist over time.

Mental Health Disorders: Mental health conditions such as depression, anxiety disorders, bipolar disorder, and schizophrenia are characterized by persistent symptoms affecting mood, cognition, behavior, and emotional well-being.

Neurological Disorders: Neurological conditions like Parkinson's disease, Alzheimer's disease, epilepsy, and migraine headaches can cause persistent symptoms affecting the brain, spinal cord, and nervous system.

Chronic Pain Syndromes: Conditions such as fibromyalgia, chronic back pain, neuropathic pain, and complex regional pain syndrome involve persistent pain that can significantly impact daily functioning and quality of life.

Cancer: Certain types of cancer, such as

leukemia, lymphoma, and metastatic cancers, may require long-term treatment and management to control the disease and prevent recurrence.

Infectious Diseases: Some infections, such as HIV/AIDS, hepatitis B and C, tuberculosis, and certain viral infections, can become chronic and require ongoing treatment and monitoring.

Management of persistent illness often involves a multidisciplinary approach, including medical treatment, medication management, lifestyle modifications, psychological support, and social interventions. Individuals living with persistent illness may face challenges related to symptom management, medication adherence, emotional well-being, social support, and maintaining quality of life.Addressing persistent illness requires a comprehensive and individualized approach that considers the specific needs, preferences, and goals of the individual. Effective management strategies focus on symptom control, preventing complications, improving function and quality of life, and supporting overall well-being. Additionally, ongoing research and advancements in medical science continue to enhance our understanding and management of persistent illness, offering hope for improved outcomes and quality of life for individuals living with these conditions.

Persistent illness can be influenced by a variety of factors, both internal and external. Some key factors contributing to persistent illness include:

Genetic Predisposition Genetic factors play an important role in making people susceptible to certain diseases. Genetic mutations or genetic disorders may increase your risk of developing chronic diseases or conditions that persist over time.

Chronic Disease Existing chronic diseases such as diabetes, high blood pressure, asthma, autoimmune diseases, and heart disease can lead to persistent diseases.

These conditions often require ongoing monitoring and treatment to control symptoms and prevent complications.

 Environmental Factors Environmental factors, such as exposure to pollutants, toxins, allergens, and infectious agents, can contribute to the development of persistent illness. Poor air quality, polluted water, exposure to harmful chemicals, and infectious diseases can negatively impact your health and cause chronic health problems.

Lifestyle Factors Unhealthy lifestyle choices such as poor diet, lack of physical activity, lack of sleep, chronic stress, substance abuse, and smoking can contribute to the onset and maintenance of the disease. These lifestyle factors can weaken the immune system, increase inflammation, and worsen chronic diseascs.

Psychological Factors Psychological factors such as chronic stress, depression, anxiety, and trauma can contribute to the development of persistent illness. Stress-related disorders, psychosomatic disorders, and mental health disorders can manifest as physical symptoms and cause lasting health problems.

Social Determinants of Health Social determinants of health, including socioeconomic status, education, employment, housing, access to health care, and social support networks, can influence disease persistence. Socioeconomic inequalities and barriers to accessing health care can exacerbate health problems and contribute to the development of chronic diseases.

Healthcare Access and Quality: Limited access to healthcare services, inadequate medical treatment, delays in diagnosis, and suboptimal management of chronic conditions can contribute to persistent illness. Inadequate healthcare resources, lack of health insurance coverage, and disparities in healthcare delivery can hinder the management and treatment of chronic health problems.

Behavioral Factors: Non-adherence to medical treatment, failure to follow recommended lifestyle modifications, and resistance to behavioral changes can contribute to the persistence of illness. Poor medication adherence, unhealthy behaviors, and reluctance to seek medical care can exacerbate health problems and lead to persistent illness.

Biological Factors Biological factors such as immune system dysfunction, hormonal imbalances, metabolic disorders, and genetic predisposition may contribute to the development of persistent diseases. Dysfunction of biological systems and imbalances in physiological processes can lead to chronic health problems that persist over time.

Complex Interactions Chronic diseases often involve complex interactions between genetic, environmental, lifestyle, psychological, social and biological factors. These multifactorial interactions contribute to disease persistence and require an integrated approach to management and treatment.

Addressing chronic disease requires a holistic approach that considers the multifaceted factors that contribute to health problems. To effectively manage and mitigate the effects of chronic disease, comprehensive management strategies that address underlying causes, promote lifestyle changes, ensure appropriate medical treatment, and address social determinants of health are essential.

Chapter 4

Mental and Emotional Well-being

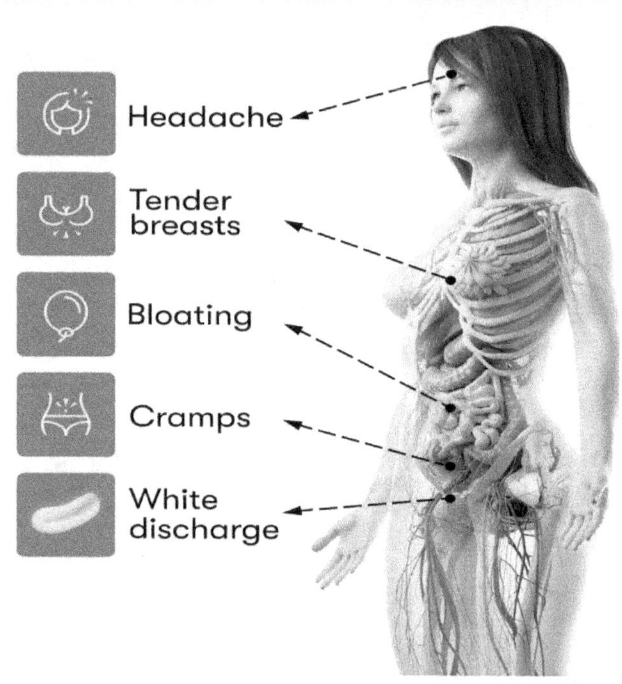

Mental well-being refers to a state of emotional, psychological, and social well-being in which an individual can cope with the normal stresses of life, work productively, maintain fulfilling relationships, and contribute to their community. It encompasses various aspects of mental health, including emotional resilience, psychological flexibility, self-esteem, positive relationships, and a sense of purpose and meaning in life.

Key components of mental well-being include:

1. Emotional Resilience:The ability to cope with adversity, stress, and challenges in a healthy and adaptive way. Individuals

with high emotional resilience can bounce back from setbacks, manage emotions effectively, and maintain a positive outlook on life.

2. Psychological Flexibility: The capacity to adapt to changing circumstances, thoughts, and emotions, allowing individuals to respond to life's challenges with openness and flexibility. Psychological flexibility involves being able to let go of unhelpful thoughts and behaviors and focus on what is meaningful and important.

3. Self-Esteem: A positive sense of self-worth and self-acceptance, characterized by confidence, self-respect, and a realistic appraisal of one's abilities and limitations.

Healthy self-esteem is essential for mental well-being and contributes to a sense of self-efficacy and empowerment.

4. Positive Relationships: Meaningful connections with others based on trust, empathy, mutual respect, and support. Strong social support networks provide emotional validation, encouragement, and a sense of belonging, which are vital for mental well-being.

5. Purpose and Meaning: A sense of purpose and direction in life, coupled with a feeling of fulfillment and satisfaction derived from meaningful activities, goals, and relationships. Having a sense of purpose contributes to a sense of identity, motivation, and overall well-being.

6. Optimism and Hope: A positive outlook on life characterized by optimism, hopefulness, and resilience in the face of adversity. Optimistic individuals are more likely to view challenges as opportunities for growth and maintain a hopeful attitude towards the future.

7. Effective Coping Strategies: Adaptive coping mechanisms and problem-solving skills that enable individuals to manage stress, regulate emotions, and navigate life's challenges effectively. Healthy coping strategies promote resilience, reduce emotional distress, and enhance overall well-being.

Promoting mental well-being involves fostering these key components through various means, including self-care practices, social support, healthy lifestyle habits, effective stress management, seeking professional help when needed, and engaging in activities that promote personal growth and fulfillment. Prioritizing mental well-being contributes to overall health, resilience, and quality of life, enabling individuals to thrive and flourish in all aspects of their lives.

Emotional well-being refers to the state of being in which an individual experiences a positive balance of emotions, effectively manages stress, and maintains healthy relationships. It encompasses various aspects of emotional health, including the ability to recognize, understand, and regulate one's emotions in a constructive manner. Emotional well-being is characterized by resilience in the face of adversity, self-acceptance, positive relationships, and overall psychological health.

Key components of emotional well-being include:

Emotional Awareness: The ability to recognize and identify one's emotions accurately, as well as understand the underlying reasons and triggers for those emotions. Emotional awareness involves being in tune with one's feelings and being able to express them in a healthy and constructive manner.

Emotional Regulation: The capacity to manage and regulate emotions effectively, including coping with stress, handling challenging situations, and modulating emotional responses. Emotional regulation involves using adaptive coping strategies to maintain emotional balance and well-being.Resilience: The ability to bounce back from setbacks, adversity, or stressful situations with strength and adaptability. Resilient individuals can cope with life's challenges, learn from setbacks, and navigate difficult circumstances with a positive attitude and outlook.

Self-acceptance: A positive self-regard and acceptance of oneself, including one's strengths, weaknesses, and imperfections.

Self-acceptance involves having a realistic and compassionate view of oneself, free from excessive self-criticism or judgment.

Healthy Relationships: Positive and supportive connections with others that provide emotional validation, empathy, and mutual respect. Healthy relationships contribute to emotional well-being by fostering a sense of belonging, security, and social support.

Stress Management: Effective coping strategies and stress management techniques that help individuals deal with life's challenges and reduce the impact of stress on their emotional well-being. This may include relaxation techniques, mindfulness practices, and seeking.

Our mental and emotional state

Mental and emotional states encompass a wide range of experiences and emotions that people may encounter in their daily lives. These conditions can fluctuate depending on a variety of factors, including environmental stimuli, personal experiences, and physiological changes. Here are some common mental and emotional conditions:

1. Happiness. It is a positive emotional state characterized by joy, contentment, and contentment. Happiness is often accompanied by feelings of happiness, gratitude, and enjoyment of life.

2. Sadness. It is an emotional state characterized by sadness, sadness, and disappointment. Grief can be caused by a variety of factors, including loss, rejection, and failure, and can vary in intensity and duration.

3. Anger: An emotional state characterized by irritation, frustration, and hostility. Anger may arise in response to a perceived threat, injustice, or violation of personal boundaries and may manifest as agitation, aggression, or anger.

4. Fear. An emotional state characterized by anxiety, anxiety, or worry about a perceived threat or danger. Fear triggers the body's fight-or-flight response, and its

intensity can range from mild anxiety to severe panic.

5. Anxiety: An emotional state characterized by excessive worry, nervousness, or fear about future events or uncertainties. Anxiety can manifest itself as physical symptoms such as rapid heartbeat, sweating, and tremors, and can interfere with daily life.

6. Stress. A mental and emotional state characterized by the body's response to perceived pressure, demand, or challenge. Stress can be caused by a variety of factors, including work, relationships, and financial issues, and can manifest as physical, emotional, and behavioral symptoms.

7. Depression. A mental health disorder characterized by persistent feelings of sadness, hopelessness, or loss of interest in activities. Depression can affect your mood, thoughts, and behavior, as well as daily functioning and quality of life.

8. Joy. It is an emotional state characterized by intense joy, excitement, and euphoria. Encouragement can be triggered by a positive event or experience and can lead to increased energy, enthusiasm, and optimism.

9. Calm. It is a mental and emotional state characterized by feelings of calmness, serenity, and relaxation. Calmness is often associated with inner peace, clarity, and emotional stability.

10. Confusion: A mental state characterized by feelings of uncertainty, disorientation, or lack of clarity. Confusion may arise in response to complex or conflicting information and can lead to difficulty in decision-making or problem-solving.

These are just a few examples of the many mental and emotional states that individuals may experience. It's important to recognize that these states are normal and can vary in intensity and duration depending on individual circumstances and coping mechanisms. Seeking support from mental health professionals or practicing self-care strategies can help individuals navigate and manage their mental and emotional states effectively.

Seeking Professional Guidance

Seeking professional guidance on living a sickness-free life is a proactive approach to maintaining optimal health and well-being. Here are some steps to consider when seeking professional guidance:

1. Primary Care Physician: Schedule regular check-ups with a primary care physician or healthcare provider to monitor your overall health, identify any potential risk factors or underlying medical conditions, and receive personalized recommendations for preventive care.

2. Health Screenings: Discuss with your healthcare provider about recommended health screenings based on your age, gender, family history, and lifestyle

factors. Medical tests, such as blood pressure tests, cholesterol tests, diabetes tests, and cancer screenings, can help identify potential health problems early.

3. Nutritionist or Dietitian: Consult with a registered dietitian or nutritionist to receive personalized diet recommendations tailored to your individual needs and health goals. A nutritionist can provide guidance on healthy eating habits, meal planning, portion control, and strategies for maintaining a balanced diet to support overall health and well-being.

4. Physical Activity Specialist: Consider working with a certified fitness trainer or physical activity specialist to develop a

personalized exercise plan that aligns with your fitness level, goals, and preferences. Regular physical activity is essential for maintaining cardiovascular health, improving strength and flexibility, and reducing the risk of chronic diseases.

5. Mental Health Professional: Seek guidance from a mental health professional, such as a psychologist, counselor, or therapist, to address any emotional or psychological challenges, stressors, or mental health concerns that may impact your overall well-being. Mental health professionals can provide support, coping strategies, and treatment options to promote emotional resilience and mental wellness.

6. Sleep Specialist: If you are experiencing a sleep disorder or having difficulty maintaining healthy sleep habits, consider consulting with a sleep specialist or medical professional who specializes in sleep medicine. A sleep specialist can evaluate your sleep patterns, identify underlying sleep disorders, and recommend steps to improve the quality and duration of your sleep.

7. Holistic Health Practitioner: Consult a holistic health professional, such as a naturopathic doctor, herbalist, or integrative medicine doctor, to learn about a holistic approach to health and wellness. Holistic health practitioners take a comprehensive approach to health,

addressing physical, mental, emotional, and spiritual aspects of well-being through a combination of conventional and alternative therapies.

8. Wellness Coach: Consider working with a certified wellness coach or health coach who specializes in supporting individuals in achieving their health and wellness goals. A wellness coach can provide guidance, accountability, and motivation to help you make sustainable lifestyle changes and adopt healthier habits for living a sickness-free life.

By seeking professional guidance from healthcare providers and wellness professionals, you can receive personalized recommendations, support, and resources to empower you in taking proactive steps towards achieving and maintaining optimal health and wellness. Remember to communicate openly with your health care team, ask questions, and become an active participant in your journey to health and wellness.

practical guidance on making lifestyle changes to support wellness

Practical guidance on making lifestyle changes to support wellness involves adopting sustainable habits and behaviors that promote physical, mental, and emotional well-being. Here are some practical steps to consider:

1. Set Specific, Realistic Goals: Identify specific wellness goals that are meaningful to you and align with your values and priorities. Make sure your goals are realistic, achievable, and measurable, and break them down into smaller, manageable steps.

2. Create a Personalized Plan: Develop a personalized wellness plan that addresses various aspects of your lifestyle, including nutrition, physical activity, sleep, stress management, and social connections. Consider consulting with a healthcare

provider, nutritionist, or wellness coach to help you create a tailored plan that meets your individual needs and goals.

3. Prioritize Nutrition: Focus on adopting a balanced and nutritious diet that includes a variety of whole foods, such as fruits, vegetables, whole grains, lean proteins, and healthy fats. Aim to minimize processed foods, sugary snacks, and unhealthy fats, and prioritize mindful eating practices, portion control, and staying hydrated.

4. Incorporate Regular Physical Activity: Find enjoyable physical activities that you can incorporate into your daily routine, such as walking, jogging, cycling, swimming, yoga, or strength training. Aim

for at least 150 minutes of moderate-intensity aerobic exercise per week, along with muscle-strengthening activities on two or more days per week.

5. Prioritize Sleep: Establish a consistent sleep schedule and prioritize getting adequate restful sleep each night. Aim for 7-9 hours of quality sleep per night, create a relaxing bedtime routine, and create a comfortable sleep environment that promotes restorative sleep.

6. Manage Stress: Practice stress-reduction techniques such as deep breathing exercises, meditation, mindfulness, progressive muscle relaxation, or yoga to manage stress effectively. Incorporate stress-relief activities into your daily

routine and prioritize self-care practices that promote relaxation and emotional well-being.

7. Cultivate Social Connections: Nurture positive relationships with family, friends, and community members by staying connected, communicating openly, and engaging in social activities. Build a support network of people who uplift and encourage you, and seek out opportunities for social connection and meaningful interactions.

8. Practice Self-Care: Prioritize self-care activities that promote physical, mental, and emotional well-being, such as taking breaks, engaging in hobbies and interests, spending time outdoors, and practicing

relaxation techniques. Set aside time for activities that bring you joy, fulfillment, and relaxation.

9. Monitor Progress and Adjust as Needed: Regularly assess your progress towards your wellness goals, celebrate your successes, and identify areas for improvement. Be flexible and willing to adjust your plan as needed based on feedback, changing circumstances, or new information.

10. Seek Support: Don't hesitate to seek support from healthcare professionals, wellness experts, or support groups if you encounter challenges or need guidance along your wellness journey. Surround yourself with a supportive community of

individuals who share your commitment to wellness and can provide encouragement, accountability, and motivation.

By implementing these practical steps and making gradual, sustainable lifestyle changes, you can support your overall wellness and cultivate a healthier, happier life. Remember that wellness is a journey, and small, consistent actions can lead to significant improvements in your physical, mental, and emotional well-being over time.

actionable steps you can take to break free from the cycle of sickness

Breaking the vicious cycle of disease requires taking proactive strategies to promote overall health and well-being. Here are actionable steps you can take to break the vicious cycle of disease:

1. Prevention comes first. Make regular appointments with your health care provider for screenings, immunizations and health assessments. Stay up to date on recommended immunizations, screenings, and preventative tests to detect and prevent potential health problems before they worsen.

2. Eat a balanced diet. Focus on eating a balanced diet rich in fruits, vegetables, whole grains, lean proteins, and healthy fats. Minimize your intake of processed foods, sugary snacks, and unhealthy fats, and prioritize mindful eating, portion

control, and hydration.

3. Include physical activity. Do regular physical activities you enjoy, such as walking, jogging, biking, swimming, or joining a group fitness class. Aim to do at least 150 minutes of moderate-intensity aerobic exercise per week and muscle-strengthening activities at least two days per week.

4. Prioritize sleep. Set a consistent sleep schedule and make it a priority to get enough restful sleep every night. Aim for 7 to 9 hours of quality sleep each night, create a relaxing bedtime routine, and create a restful sleep environment that promotes restorative sleep.

5. Stress Management: To effectively

manage stress, practice stress-reduction techniques such as deep breathing exercises, meditation, mindfulness, progressive muscle relaxation, or yoga. Incorporate stress-relieving activities into your daily routine and prioritize self-care practices that promote relaxation and emotional well-being.

6. Practice good hygiene Practice good hygiene, including washing hands regularly with soap and water, practicing appropriate food handling and hygiene, and maintaining clean personal spaces and environments. These methods help prevent the spread of infectious diseases and diseases.

7. Avoid Harmful Substances: Limit or avoid excessive consumption of alcohol,

tobacco, and illicit drugs, as they can weaken the immune system, impair organ health, and increase susceptibility to infections, respiratory problems, and chronic diseases.

8. Seek Mental Health Support: Prioritize your mental and emotional well-being by seeking support from mental health professionals, counselors, or support groups if you experience symptoms of stress, anxiety, depression, or other mental health concerns. Practice self-care activities that promote emotional resilience and well-being.

9. Build a support network. Surround yourself with a support network of family, friends, and community members who encourage and encourage you. Develop

positive relationships and meaningful relationships with others who share your values and support your health goals.

10. Educate yourself. Stay up-to-date on health topics, preventative measures, and evidence-based health promotion strategies. Expand your knowledge and make informed decisions about your health with trusted sources of health information, educational resources, and medical experts. By taking proactive steps to prioritize your health and wellbeing, you can break the cycle of illness and live a healthier, happier life. Remember that small, consistent actions can significantly improve your overall health and well-being over time.

Why
AM I ALWAYS SICK
Breaking the habits
Unvailing The
Mystery Of
Getting
Unneccessary
Sick
BY
Dr Sebastian Wayne

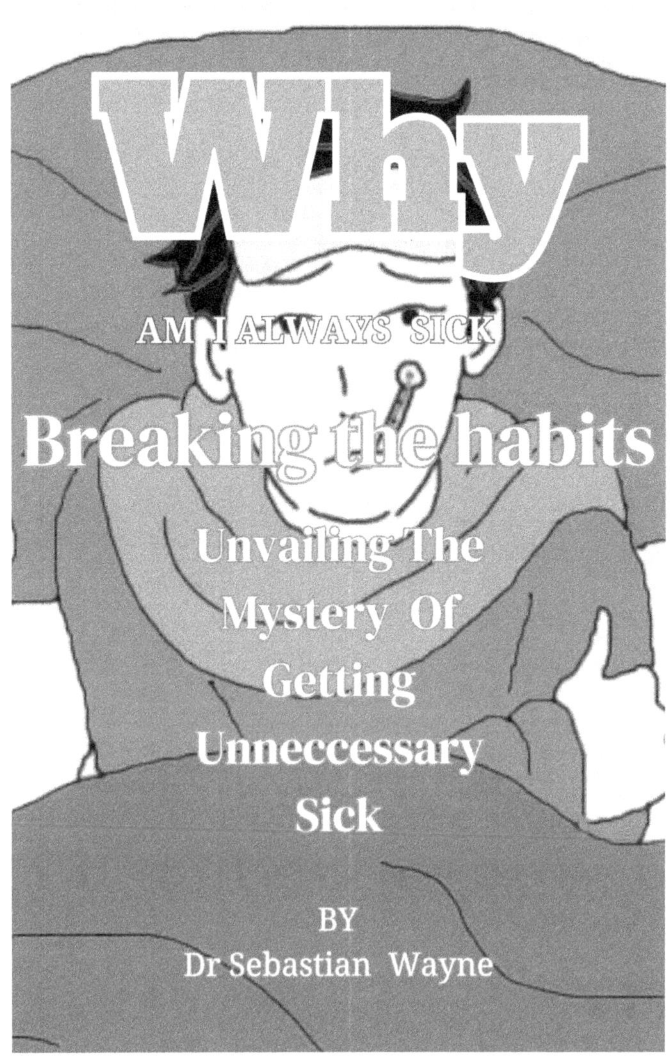

168

www.ingramcontent.com/pod-product-compliance
Lightning Source LLC
Chambersburg PA
CBHW070949250726
48663CB00002B/142